# The No-Diet Lifestyle

Victor R. Pierson, III

Printed in the United States of America

ISBN-13: 978-1481255974

ISBN-10: 1481255975

*To Audrey*

# CONTENTS

# Special Thanks

Chas Minor and Jenni Mills

Cover Photo - Randi Caylor

This book would have never been written if it were not for the support of my dear friends in *The Weekly Game Plan* group on Facebook. Thank you so much for bucking me up when I was low and disillusioned and for cheering me through the good times.

Your friendship and support has meant the world to me and I could never have completed this book without you.

# Introduction

For years, friends have asked me for my recipe for this or that after eating a dish I had prepared and I would look at them like a deer caught in the headlights. I would simply say that I would get back to them and then conveniently forget.

Once on Facebook, however, I couldn't seem to get away from the queries and I finally told the truth as to why I was so reluctant to reveal my secrets. I explained that most of my recipes were for one serving and based on a system designed to work within the structure of a restaurant kitchen, my main employment for over thirty-five years. To my amazement, this did not stop the requests. People were looking for these kinds of recipes, especially new empty-nesters and those who were single. After much nudging, I agreed to write a cookbook explaining the system and releasing the recipes to the world.

I've always had issues with my heft. I have tried every diet that was ever put out including my doctor's little booklet that proved what an austere diet looked like. Every time I got to my goal weight, I reached for whatever was denied me for the entire time and gained all the weight back. In most cases, I gained even more weight than I had lost. Finally I decided that enough was enough and vowed never to go on another diet again.

About three months into working on the book, a friend came over to pick up some vegetables from my garden. He look at me in astonishment and said it looked like I had lost some weight. I told him that my clothes did seem a bit loose, but being in pants with draw strings and triple extra large shirts, I wasn't quite sure. I knew I had more energy because to clear my mind after writing all morning, I started taking a walk.

I have never been what you would call a couch potato; I'm more of a computer spud. Sitting at the computer all day and chowing down on whatever was quick and easy, eating it at the computer and no exercise, I was more of a slug than anything else.

However, when I starting writing the book, I started using the system I was writing about and all the computer snacking came to a halt. Limited on food dollars, I simply did not have the funds for both snacks and the good food I was preparing. When my friend left, I eagerly jumped on the scale and realized I had lost 35 pounds.

I remember just standing there, not only happy, but a bit puzzled as to how I lost the weight. I decided to start a journal to keep track of everything I was eating and to record the amount of exercise I was getting. I found that I was eating a lot of fresh vegetables and fruit that I grew in my back yard, supplemented with fresh food on sale at my local green grocer. As the need arose, I found myself walking more and more until I needed some transportation to get to other parts of the county, where a bus would have taken me all day to travel to and from. It was at that time, a friend was kind enough to let me borrow his bicycle.

Riding the bicycle was the best thing. I could now easily go to the post office, the grocery store and get home without it taking all day and feeling great to boot! I would ride at least every other day, most days without a destination, but just to have the wonderful, stress-free hour to clear the kinks in my mind.

Keeping that journal for two months gave me great insight into how I lost the weight, and I began to feel that this book had a greater purpose than to share some recipes.

# The Ride of a Lifetime

There came a time in writing the book when I became disillusioned and stopped writing. Earlier versions of the book confused those who were proof reading it for me. I was stumped as to what I needed to do to make the method of cooking clearer. I had taught people the system one-on-one, but writing was a new form of presentation and I was apprehensive using this medium. I went into a re-write mode, but soon had total writer's block.

On October 17, 2012, I embarked on a trip on my bike that I did not have on any 'Bucket List, nor any desire to do before. I mounted my bicycle at Young Circle on US 1 in Hollywood, Florida and headed south. I decided to ride my bicycle to Mile Marker Zero, located in Old Town Key West, Florida. Since I did not do any special training for this ride, I took my time, three and a half days, spending 22 hours 27 minutes of actual travel time to complete the 185.19-mile trek. It was on this trip that I realized that at the age of 57, I was no longer a *Computer Slug* and that was the main purpose of this book.

The original book had grown into a 255-recipe book with many variations, but without direction. It was at that point I decided to focus more on the nutritional aspects and cooking method without the extended and complete cookbook. I realize that this system may not be for everyone and many may not see the results I did, but I still feel it was worth it to share exactly what I did.

This book includes a sample of the system to get you started. The complete cookbook will be released at a later time to give the reader more options and variety.

# Chapter 1: The Basics

## My Daily Nutritional Plan

In the course of writing this book, the USDA's MyPyramid was replaced by a new program called MyPlate. While MyPlate is more representative of what your balanced diet should look like, it fails to take into consideration the realistic approach I took, not to mention the fact that no one has yet to put what we eat into precise categories. Unless you are a nutritionist, some of the recommendations are just plain confusing, such as one question I had that was never answered: "When is a Navy Bean considered a vegetable and when is it considered a protein?"

So, let us simplify all of this government mumbo-jumbo and go back to basics. Let us keep our portions to a normal size, keep to the amount of servings of a well rounded lifestyle, and get some exercise to burn the energy our food gives us.

After keeping a food journal, once I realized I was losing weight, I started researching the nutritional properties of the food I was consuming. While I did not adjust what I was doing, the research showed me why I was losing the weight. I stuck with what I was doing and realized, once I got down to a weight I was comfortable with, that I only had to adjust one food group (Starch) to maintain my weight.

The following food groups are what I used to lose and maintain my weight and overall nutrition:

## 4 servings of Vegetables

All servings of vegetables are measured when raw. If vegetables are used from a can or commercially frozen, use the serving size stated on the packaging. I find it is best to have at least one serving each of green leafy vegetables, orange vegetables, tomatoes and squash. The use of homemade vegetable juice and vegetable stock in your mixes and recipes add to the nutritional values to your food.

What are not considered vegetables in my nutritional plan are white potatoes, peas, corn, beets and yucca. See Starches for more information.

You should always try to use fresh, however, if fresh is not available, use dried or frozen. Avoid canned if all possible. My only exception to the can rule are sardines and pineapple that is packed in juice.

Rule of thumb: A serving of green, leafy vegetables is two handfuls; A serving of all other vegetables is one handful.

## *4 servings of Fruit*

I love fruit, especially fresh fruit. No fruit is out of bounds, however, canned fruit is usually not used due to added sugars. A serving of fruit is one handful, or a medium sized fruit. A whole banana is fine, if it is no more than five inches in length. I'm forever grabbing a handful of grapes for a snack.

Dry fruits are very good as well. You should always eat at least one serving of fruit a day that is high in fiber, such as figs or prunes.

## *3 servings of Whole Grain*

Whole grains give you the over all fiber you need in your diet. Breads made with over processed flour, such as white wheat flour and corn meal are not in this group. Neither are rice and pasta. See Starch.

Wild rice, whole grain cereals and my favorite, Buckwheat Groats are excellent choices of Whole Grain.

A serving of Whole Grain is one slice of bread. See packaging for serving sizes for cereals, groats and rice.

## *3 servings of Dairy*

Dairy is very important, and as we age, is the most ignored. If you are a Vegan, please make sure you take supplements to ensure you are getting the proper amount of calcium.

Milk and cheese are great choices, but don't over do. A serving of cheese is one ounce. Not sure how much that is? Purchase an 8-ounce block of cheese and divide it into 8 pieces. If it helps, do that every time you purchase cheese.

## 3 servings of Protein

Beans, fish, meat, seeds, nuts and poultry are good sources of protein, needed to ensure that your blood stays healthy. The most important thing to remember in the group is serving sizes and preparation methods.

Due to food allergies, I stayed clear of nuts, however, I mainly used beans and fish, eating meat and poultry only once or twice a week. This was a choice because of the tight budget I was on.

Alternative methods were used to cook my protein, such as poaching poultry in vegetable stock and slow cooking meats. A serving of meat and poultry is 3 ounces. A serving of fish and other seafood is 4 ounces. A serving of beans is one handful. All servings are based on raw weights. Any fats and oils used to cook your protein comes from the next group, Oily.

## 2.5 servings of Oily

In cooking savory foods, I only use Extra Virgin Olive Oil. Don't skimp, buy the best! I have always liked olive oil for its flavor, so, it was a no-brainer for me. I also use butter. Simple ingredients rule: chemical ingredients cannot be good for you, period.

Serving size is that which is on the packaging. The serving size is for what is consumed, not what is used. For example, if you used olive oil to sauté vegetables, but only added the vegetables leaving oil in the pan, the total serving would be measured as 1/2.

Word of warning: do not substitute oils, fat and butter in the recipes; they may not turn out as they should.

## 1.5 servings of Starch

The Starch Group is the only group where the number of servings can change periodically. This group gives your body energy to do the things you physically do. If you are losing weight, your body has already stored a lot of the starches you need, so, do not increase the amount of servings. However, once you have reached your goal weight, without downsizing the amount of daily exercise, you can increase your starches by one half serving.

People who start training for extended activities such as running in marathons and do not want to lose weight and/or do not want to run out of energy, should increase the servings of starch to 4 or 5 servings. Once you have completed such activity or decrease your extra activity, you should lower your servings back down to 2 servings.

My first December after I lost my weight, I went to parties and was given my favorite, Chocolate Fudge, for Christmas. I did not decrease or increase my activity, and as a result, gained eight pounds; a small weight gain compared to previous years. In January, I decreased my starches back to the 1.5 servings level and lost the weight I had gained the month before in only three weeks. I then changed my starch servings to two and continued to maintain my new normal weight.

Funny thing about Starches ... there are two types: Good Starches and Bad Starches.

Let us talk about the Bad Starches first. Bad starches should be used sparingly as most of them are void of nutritional value. The following are bad starches, listed with the worse offenders first:

- All alcohol beverages
- Sugar based sodas
- Candy
- Brown sugar
- Granulated and powdered sugar
- Honey
- Corn
- Green Peas
- Yucca
- Beets
- Any food not listed that your doctor specifically wants you to avoid

Good starches are best used to increase your energy for extended physical activity. These good starches are:

- White rice
- Pasta
- White wheat flour, used in biscuits & white bread

- Cornmeal
- White and Red potatoes
- Black eyed peas
- Corn-based cereals

## *1 serving of Dessert*

An earlier draft of this book had the subtitle: A Realistic Approach to American Cooking. I've always felt that my earlier downfall to losing and maintaining my weight was the innate 'going on a diet' approach of denying me of the foods I loved the most. The majority of these foods were desserts. Thinking of a realist approach to a lifetime way of eating also had to include dessert. This serving does not count against any other group. I just made sure the serving size was of normal proportion and if I did have a super-duper dessert, it would only be once a week. Don't deny yourself of a little indulgence now and then!

### Serving Sizes

This brings us to an important question: What *exactly* is a serving size?

Since no foods are off limits, I am reminded of my remote youth. I have an old *Pepsi* bottle that brags that unlike their competitor, *Coca-Cola*, for the same price, this bottle has "Two Servings." It is a 12-ounce bottle. Back then, there were only one size served in restaurants. If you ordered a cola, you would have been served a 10-ounce glass, filled with ice and six ounces of soda. That soda was also considered a treat, not an every day beverage; we had water for that.

Through shrewd marketing, over time, we have gone from that normal size to medium, large, extra large, jumbo, super size, etc. The same goes for our food consumption over the coarse of the last 50 years. Even the size of our plates are two to three inches in diameter larger than their 1950's counterparts. Ever gone into an old, un-remodeled home and found that the kitchen cabinets are too shallow for your dinner plates to fit? It isn't because they built on the cheap in the early part of the 20th century; it is because of our increasing obsession for bigger is better.

We no longer know what a proper serving size is due to commercial propaganda to get us to buy more than what we need. It has caused us to get into a habit that is very hard to break, especially if we have never known anything else. Rather than go through psychotherapy to break this consumption habit, we can control over-eating and over-preparing by changing the things we eat off of and the cooking vessels we use on a day-to-day basis.

We so often cook and serve to the size of the dish or pot we are using, resulting in preparing too much food. To prevent this from happening, it is a wise move to use dishes and cooking vessels that are more in line with the amount of food we need. What I use personally, are the following.

- 10 oz soufflé cup with optional lid, oven/freezer/micro safe
- 14 oz au gratin dish, round or oval, oven/freezer/micro safe

- 8-inch dinner plate (not counting the rim)
- 10-ounce bowl (aka cereal bowl)
- 4-oz "Monkey Dish"
- 8-in cast iron skillet
- 1-qt and 2-qt sauce pan
- 1.5 qt Slow Cooker
- Mortar and Pestle

The dishes can be usually found cheaply at yard sales and on eBay. The cooking vessels and appliances are relatively inexpensive due to their size. As you use the recipes in this book, you will learn what a serving size is.

# Food Procurement

What is it that every restaurant is trying to do? It is trying to make money. This is done in several ways that are not unlike the things that people do at home. Food wholesalers promote their products with sales, much like grocers do. They also have introduction prices and incentives to get the restaurant's Food and Beverage manager to purchase and try out their new products, including offering samples. The manufacturers and providers of food aimed at the home buyer do the same thing by offering coupons and free samples.

So, already, we can see how our home opportunities to save money are very much like the opportunities for a restaurant. The only difference in the two is with a restaurant, the money they save goes toward their profit line; for the private sector, the money saved can go to other expenses in the home and the opportunity to save money to do more enjoyable things.

But I am going to go another step further, the step that all restaurant managers know, but have never told the general public. There are four general rules for keeping your food costs down, and over time, you will see the overall quality of your food improve, while the cost of your food lowers.

General rules for keeping your food costs down:

1. Get in the habit of using all parts of the fresh meats and produce that you purchase. You have paid good money for these, especially if you paid for them 'by the pound' so, it just stands to reason that if you throw anything away that could be used for something else, you are in essence throwing your hard-earned money away. Suggestions, tips and instructions for this rule are located throughout this book.

2. Home grow at least one item that you eat. Not everyone has the space, time, ability or experience to have full-fledged gardens, however, just growing one thing will bring freshness to your table at the lowest possible cost. Suggestions and instructions will be included later in this book.

3. Buy produce locally. Not only will it help your local economy, it will allow you to meet the people who grow your food. They can answer questions regarding pesticides, growing seasons and preparation tips. You can also ask them about other produce you might be interested in. Farmers want to grow what their customers need, but the

farmer cannot read your mind. If you don't ask, it will never be available. If you can find a couple of friends who have been looking for the same item, get together at the market and I'm sure the farmer will try a small plot to see if you really will buy it. Farmers are very willing to work with their customers, so talk to them.

4. Get to know your butcher. Not everything your grocer has is displayed in the refrigerated bins out front. If you are looking for something, ask the butcher. In fact, tell your butcher what it is you're making. All butchers have their cheapest cuts and scraps in the back and will gladly get them for you. These items are usually cheaper year round without a sale. Knowing your butcher will also help you to get the kind of cut you want from what is out front. If you do not feel comfortable deboning a chicken or you need ground pork, lamb, or veal, ask your butcher to do it for you. There is usually no extra cost for this.

In addition to these general rules, I would add these:

• Make a rough draft of your weekly menu and take inventory of what you have on hand. Using that information, make a list of everything you need before going to the market. People for years have forgotten these lists and run amok in the store, over bought and ended up spending more money in gas and time to make smaller trips back to the store for things they *really* need. Thanks to modern technology, it should be easier to make sure you have the list on you. I'm sure there is an App for that.

• Unless you are cooking for four or more, buying in bulk will not save you money unless you have an effective storage system. Suggestions on storage will be discussed later in this book.

• Make a budget and stick to it. This might take some time as you figure out just how much you need and how much you can afford to feed yourself.

> 1. Do not include cleaning supplies, paper goods and pet food in your food budget. Even if you buy them in the same store, these things need to go in their own categories in your budget.

> 2. Do include one-time use items used in storage such as aluminum foil, plastic wrap, zipper-style plastic bags and seal-a-meal style film and bags.

# Low Cost, High Quality

In the course of providing yourself with the highest quality of food while keeping to your budget, it is imperative that you do at least one of the following:

• Purchase veggies from a farmer's market weekly.
• Grow at least one thing you use in the kitchen.

In this section, we will be talking about the latter, as buying locally has already been discussed.

No matter where you live, you can grown at least one thing that you will use regularly in your kitchen and/or at the table. While these ideas are listed very basically in this book, I would suggest further research at your local library will give you more detail and recommendations for your particular living quarters.

No matter where you live, or what type of item you decide to grow, you will produce more than you need. Take the time to share your harvest with a friend.

1. **Apartments/Condos** *with no patio or balcony that has very little natural light*: Ha! thought you were off the hook, eh? Well, here are three ideas for you.

> a. **Grow alfalfa, mung beans, or soybeans sprouts**. I use a sprouter that I bought for $10 and I can make three batches at a time. It is quite simple. Soak the seeds for 10-18 hours in water. Drain and cover. Wash the seeds at least twice a day, however more is better. You can wash the seed up to eight times a day. You repeat this for three to four days and then set the sprouts near a window (does not have to be direct sunlight) to 'green up'. Rinse again, drain very well, and store in the refrigerator in a storage container. I use mainly alfalfa sprouts for salads, sometimes just grabbing a handful for a snack. Mung bean sprouts are great for a stir fry. $10 of seeds, if you grow every week, will last 1 year.

> b. **Grow Mushrooms**. This may take a bit of research before you try, but if you have a dark, cool spot in your home, this might be something

you can successfully grow. You can even grow mushrooms in spent coffee grounds.

c. **Hydroponics**. This is 21st Century crop growing for your home. Using controlled lighting and a liquid nutrient growing medium, you'll be able to grow herbs, cherry tomatoes and assorted leaf lettuce. There are currently several hydroponic appliances on the market and they can be quite expensive if you don't use them on a regular basis. Try to find one that lets you buy your own seeds.

2. **Apartments and Condos** *with patios, balconies and /or natural light*

a. You can do what those with little or no natural light do PLUS

b. Using self-watering pots on your patio is your best bet if you are first starting out. There are many kinds of potting soil available. Get a potting soil that has nutrients already formulated into the soil. Ask your local garden center for help.

3. **Homes & Townhomes/Townhouses**

In addition to what has been discussed for other home types, you have the ability to try these other methods.

a. Try adding herbs to your flower beds. Herbs can be a nice addition to any flower bed offering a variation of color with their many shades of green. Most herbs can become quite tall, so they make great foundation plants. If allowed to bolt, the seeds will fall to the ground and you can get a couple of years of herbs with just one planting. Plant your seeds indoors and once your herbs have formed 5-9 leaves and frost is no longer a worry, plant outdoors.

b. If you think you are ready to think bigger, try a small three-foot by three-foot raised bed or a 48-inch raised round bed in your backyard. Your raised bed should be built with materials that can withstand moisture, sunlight and are resistant to molds and insects. Do not use pressure treated wood, as such wood contains harmful chemicals that will contaminate your veggies and will make you very, very ill. It is best to purchase cedar or go with a kit that can be found at any garden store or online. I have included the beds that I use on my website. Included here are my main suggestions:

- The easiest starter garden is what I call *The Salad Bowl*. It is a 48-inch round raised bed in which I sow assorted greens and bib lettuce. My favorite lettuce mix is Mesclun Mix and I also like to plant some mustard greens for variety.

- The next raised bed you might want to try is the 3x3 foot bed. This bed should be at least 10-inches deep. You can plant something different in each square foot. For example, in each square foot, you could plant the following:

| 2<br>Basil | 9<br>Shallots | 1 Hot<br>Pepper |
|---|---|---|
| 1 Cherry<br>Tomato | 1 Beefsteak<br>Tomato | 1 Plum<br>Tomato |
| 4<br>Cilantro | 1 Bell<br>Pepper | 5 Swiss<br>Chard |

# For heaven's sake, don't kill your diners!

It is very important to keep in mind the basics of good habits when it comes to food safety through proper food handling, preparation and storage. Please keep these simple rules in mind.

## Keep hot food hot; Keep cold food cold

Your refrigerator should have a constant temperature range of 35 to 40 degrees F. Keeping a refrigerator thermometer in your refrigerator is a great idea so you can check the current temperature on a regular basis. Extremely perishable foods, such as milk and mayonnaise must be kept at these temperatures and should be discarded if allowed to warm up above these temperatures before consuming. Don't take a chance.

Your freezer should not reach a temperature above zero degrees Fahrenheit. A hanging freezer thermometer is very helpful to determining whether or not your freezer is set correctly.

Hot foods should be kept hot on the stove, held hot over steam or over flame burners such as chafing fuel. Once you have served your food, any leftovers should be placed in a clean container, dated and immediately placed in the refrigerator or freezer.

## Food Rotation

Make sure all your prepared food is labeled and dated. Use the oldest first.

## Keep All Surfaces Clean

I use the *bucket method* of keeping my surfaces clean. Inexpensive microfiber cloths are available at your local home improvement store and I find that they are the best. They usually come in packs of twenty-five. Use the cloths once and throw in a bucket. If the cloths are extremely soiled, then launder them. Otherwise, fill the bucket with hot, soapy water and add 2 T of bleach per gallon. Let them sit submerged for 15-20 minutes and then rinse. Wring out access water and fold damp if you are going to use them immediately, otherwise, either throw them in the dryer or hang them outside to dry.

## Ban Pets From Kitchen Surfaces

Pets should not be allowed to touch surfaces in your kitchen. **PERIOD!!**

## Cross-contamination Can and Will *Kill* You.

Be aware that cross-contamination is one of the major problems in any kitchen. Do not allow cooked food to come in contact with uncooked food. Each type of food should have its own cutting surface. Turning a cutting surface over DOES NOT prevent cross-contamination.

Every kitchen should have a cutting board for each of the following: Raw Meat, Raw Poultry, Raw Seafood, Raw Pork, Raw Vegetables and one for cooked food.

## Jars, baggies and old butter tubs, OH MY!

When it comes to basic storage of food, it is real simple. Use one or more of the following methods:

- Place food in a food storage bag manufactured with a closer and designed for refrigerator or freezer storage.
- Use a vacuum sealer system available commercially.
- Place food in a clean, sterilized glass jar with a tight fitting lid. Remember, if the food you are storing is acidic, you should always use glass for storage.
- Dry goods should be stored in containers with lids that seal out bugs and moisture. Some foods require less light and should be placed in tinted glass.
- Use any plastic container with a tight fitting lid that has the NSF mark on it or was on the packaging it came in. These plastic containers have been designed to be washed, sanitized

and reused. If you do not hear a pop or snap when you close the lid, then try another lid. If you still do not hear it, then your container/lid has a flaw and it should only be used for non-food items or recycled.

Never use any plastic bag twice nor any tub or container that you purchased with food in it. These items cannot be thoroughly washed and cannot be sanitized adequately to store your food. These items, if used again, will cause bacteria to form in places that are impossible to clean and will make you sick.

No arguments on this issue, I don't care if your mother did it, your grandmother did it or your cousin Vicki did it: **DO NOT USE PLASTIC BUTTER TUBS, MILK JUGS OR COTTAGE CHEESE CONTAINERS THAT YOU BOUGHT AT THE STORE.** These containers were made just seconds before they were filled with the food product you purchased and designed for one-time use only. Recycle or use them in your workshop or craft room.

# Chapter 2: The Method

The core of this method is to prepare nutritious food quickly and conveniently by using vegetable, fruit and dry mixes that you prepare yourself. With these mixes, not only will you save money, but you will also have total control over what goes into your food.

Having this total control, you will never have to worry about you or anyone you cook for accidentally consuming a food item that they are allergic to. Some of these mixes will only have to be prepped once or twice a year; other mixes will have to be prepped weekly. You should never have to prep more than an hour a week, unless you're planning a dinner party for more than your usual number of servings per meal.

Most of the recipes in this book are for one serving. However, the ones that make more than one serving will provide an explanation how it adds to your advantage. With this system in place, you will never make too much or too little. This also prevents two main problems people have:

Over eating occurs when too much food is prepared. Serving the right amount of any dish will assist you in losing and maintaining your ideal weight.

Wasted food is the number one reason people have trouble keeping within their food budget. This method eliminates what I call 'push-back' leftovers. These leftovers are put in the refrigerator, pushing older leftovers to the rear of the refrigerator. These 'push-back' leftovers invariably end up in the trashcan, usually after taking on a new life of their own (mold).

To make more than one serving, you simply multiply the number of servings to create up to four servings. If you are using the suggested cooking dishes and pans, you can make more without having to modify the recipe using the original formulas.

# Cooking with Formulas

Most of the recipes originally contained ingredient formulas that allowed me to adjust ingredients to produce dishes for larger quantities of the dish. While these formulas are great to produce these same recipes for large groups of people such as a dinner party or to carry it to a potluck dinner, they are beyond the scope of this book.

All formulas have been removed from the recipes in this book, as this book is meant to be used by households cooking for 1 to 4 people. For further information on how to use formulas, please consult "The No-Diet Lifestyle Cookbook, Unabridged" where the subject is explained in detail.

# Prep Your Food for Convenience

Busy lives and busy schedules command a food preparation method that reduces the cooking time to produce the best nutritious solution for any household. Commercial companies know that. They make and sell food products to help speed up the cooking process, however, as the last fifty years have shown, these heavily marketed products have ingredients that may not be as healthy and nutritious as they should be.

I have a saying: "If you cannot pronounce an ingredient or you do not know what an ingredient is, do not put it in your mouth!" Flavor enhancers, food coloring, extra and unneeded salt and sugar, artificial flavors, artificial colors, preservatives and other chemicals in these mixes do not add to the nutritional needs of your family, and in many cases can do more harm than good.

# When and How to Prep

Soon after putting your food away when you return home from the grocery store or farmer's market, you should take inventory of the mixes you have on hand and decide which mixes you need to prep. These mixes will save you time as you prepare your meals and your family is staring you down with that hungry look in their eyes.

Your mixes should be stored in a clean, clear container with a tight-fitting lid, that you have washed and sanitized. Line the bottom of your container with dry terry cloth or paper towel. Remember to never add new mix to old mix. If you have older mix, use that first and use a fresh container.

Place chopped vegetables and fruit in a large mixing bowl and mix completely. Then transfer your mix into the prepared container. Top your vegetable mixes with a paper towel and place an ice cube on top. Add an additional ice cube every time you use your mix, draining excess water, if needed.

Make sure to label the container with the name of the mix and the date you prepared it. Vegetable mixes and Fruit mixes containing fresh fruit should not be held for more than seven days.

Vegetable and Fruit mixes contain a ratio for measurement instead of a quantity. It is up to you to decided how much you will need. A ratio of 1:1 is equal parts of all ingredients. A ratio of 2:1 would be two parts of the first ingredient listed and one part of the second ingredient. For example, if you know you are going to need 3 cups of a mix that has a ratio of 2:1 and the list of ingredients is onions and green peppers, in that order, you would need to prep 2 cups of onion and 1 cup of green peppers.

## *Chop Sizes*

I use three simple and basic chop sizes:

**Finely chopped**: Vegetable and Fruit that are 1/8 inch or smaller. Mixes that are finely chopped are used in recipes such as Tuna Salad, Salmon Cakes and Meatloaf.

**Coarsely chopped**: Vegetable and Fruit that are cut 1/4- to 1/2-inch. Mixes that are coarsely chopped are used for incorporating into salads such as a Green Leafy, Potato, and Pasta. They are also used in some soups and fruit pies.

**Chunk-a Chunk-a**: Vegetable and Fruit that are cut 1/2- to 1-inch. Mixes that contain this cut are used for side dishes, soups, pot pies, cobblers, and stews.

I also use these specialty cuts occasionally:

**Coin Cut, regular**: This cut pertains to eggplant, zucchini, yellow squash, cucumbers, tomatoes, carrots, onions, most root vegetables and most fruit. This cut will produce a round slice that is at least 1/4-inch in width.
**Coin Cut, shaved**: This cut is the same as a **Coin Cut, regular**, but is less than 1/4-inch thick.

**Half Moon, regular**: This cut starts out as a Coin **Cut, regular,** but then is cut in half, producing a half moon or crescent shape.

**Half Moon, shaved**: This cut is the same as a **Half Moon, regular**, but is less than 1/4-inch thick.

**Rings, thick**: This cut pertains mainly to onions and peppers. A **Rings, thick** slice is 1/4- to 1/2-inch. Such a cut would be used to make onion rings or produce raw onions and peppers for a salad.

**Rings, thin**: This cut is just like **Rings, thick**, but cut less than 1/4-inch thick. Such cuts would be used, for example, in French Onion Soup or for sautéed onions for steak subs.

# Terminology Used in Mixes and Recipes

**Serving**: The amount of food served to each diner.

**A/P Flour**: All Purpose Flour

**H**: A handful of an ingredient that is measured by filling your hand that is cupped, as if drinking water from your hand.

**P**: A Pinch. A pinch is a quarter to a half of 1/8 teaspoon.

**Splash or Dollop**: A Splash and a Dollop are very similar in that both amounts are at the discretion of the cook. A Splash is in reference to liquids, usually 1 ounce or less; a Dollop is in reference to a solid, such as sour cream.

**t**: A level teaspoon

**T**: A level tablespoon

**C**: A level U.S. Standard cup measure.

# The Mixes

If you are not sure how much of each chop size you need, make more of the Chunk-a Chunk-a, as you can always make it smaller with a couple of shots in the food processor.

## Fresh Vegetable Mixes

<u>All-American Trinity Mix</u>
1:1:1
Yellow Onion
Celery
Sweet Pepper, any color or mixed

<u>Cool Summer Mix</u>
1:1
Scallions (include 2-3 inches of green leaves)
Celery

<u>Mirepoix</u>
1:1:1
Onions
Carrots
Celery

# Fruit Mixes

Golden Fruit Mix (cut only as directed here)
2:1:1
Golden Delicious Apples, cored, coarsely chopped
Golden Raisins, whole
White Seedless Grapes, sliced in half

**Note:** Dip apples in a solution of 1:2 lemon juice :
water, to prevent apples from turning brown.

Savory Dried Fruit Mix
1:1:1:1
Golden Raisins
Dried Apricots
Dried Pineapple
Sun Dried or Dehydrated Tomatoes

**Note:** Cut everything the same size as the raisins and
store in an air-tight container in a cool, dark place.

# PREP MIXES

Some complex recipes have steps that are actually full recipes within a recipe. When such recipes are called for in more than one recipe, or are seldom, if ever, served on their own, I refer to them as *Prep Mixes*.

These Prep Mixes may contain other fresh or Prep Mixes, but should really be done in advance. Most of the following mixes need time for their flavors to 'marry' and age, but still will be considered as fresh.

Some are available commercially, but if you are trying to stay away from chemicals and preservatives in your food or you have food allergy concerns, then these mixes are surely to be popular and in reality, a necessity.

## Baking and Flour-based

Egg Mix
6 whole large eggs OR 4 large egg whites
2 T water

1. Beat until smooth, silky, and one color. The mix should have no bubbles.
2. Store in a clean, air-tight container in the refrigerator for no more than seven days.

**Note:** You can substitute Egg Mix with a commercial egg substitute such as Egg Beaters.

## Egg Wash

1:2 Egg Mix : milk (1% fat or more, do not use skim milk)

Stir milk and Egg Mix. Mix should not be foamy. Use a pastry brush to apply.

Mix should be kept in a glass container and refrigerated for no more than seven days.

## Pie Pastry

2 C A/P flour OR 1 C A/P flour + 1 C whole wheat
   flour
1 t table salt
3/4 C shortening, vegetable, solid (do not use oil)
1/2 C very cold water

1.  In a large bowl, sift together flour and salt.
2.  Using a pastry cutter or fork, blend in shortening until mixture is coarse, like corn meal. I usually end up using my hands to ensure the shortening is well incorporated in the flour.
3.  Add the cold water and stir with fork until the dough forms a ball and is no longer sticky. Do not over mix.
4.  Divide dough in half.
5.  On a floured surface, roll out dough to 1/8-inch thickness.
6.  For a bottom crust, cut 1-inch larger than the top of your pie plate, au gratin dish or tart pan and press dough into the plate. For a top crust, using the top of the intended dish as a guide, cut the same size as the dish; using a thimble, cut out the center to allow for venting.

If you are making top crusts for future use, place on a cookie tray and freeze. Take out frozen pastry crusts, place a sheet of waxed paper between each and put into a ziplock freezer bag, pressing out extra air. Return to freezer.

If you are in need of a pre-baked pie shell, prick holes on the bottom and sides with a fork and place pastry beads to weigh down pastry. Bake in a 450°F oven for 10-12 minutes.

**Note:** Like biscuits, pie pastry will be tough if worked too much. If you want flakey crust, knead as little as possible.

## Self-rising Flour

1 C A/P flour
1/2 t table salt
1 1/2 t baking powder

Sift together all ingredients and mix completely. Place in a tightly covered container.
Yield=1 C

## Vanilla Sugar

2 vanilla beans, whole or scraped
4 C sugar, granulated

1. Slice vanilla beans lengthwise and scape seeds of one bean into an airtight container filled with the sugar.
2. Mix well.

3.  Scrape the other bean into a freezer container or vacuum storage bag and place in your freezer for later use.
4.  Bury both bean pods into the sugar and seal tightly.
5.  Let sit for two weeks.
6.  Remove bean pods, wipe off sugar and freeze for later use, as you can use them to make more sugar for up to three times.
7.  Use like regular sugar.

## Yellow Cake Mix; Complete

6 C self-rising cake flour
4 C Vanilla Sugar
1 1/2 C pure vegetable shortening (not oil)
6 T Pasteurized Dried Whole Eggs
1 1/8 C Nido Full Cream Milk Powder

1.  Cut shortening into flour until you have a texture of corn meal.
2.  Stir in remaining ingredients until thoroughly mixed.
3.  Place into an airtight container.
4.  Will keep for eight months in a cool, dark place or in the freezer.

# Back Burner Stock Pot and Soup Prep

The Back Burner Stock Pot system enables you to stretch your food dollar and nutritional balance by using food parts and pieces that most cooks throw in the trash. By using scraps from peeling and cleaning vegetables, you can make your own fresh and nutrient-filled stock.

While there are quite a few types of stock pots you can use, in this book, we will only be using Vegetable Stock. To start with a base stock:

Place in a pot, 3 C Mirepoix Mix and 2 C of Cool Summer Mix, Chunk-a Chunk-a, and cover with water. Simmer for four hours, stirring occasionally. Strain out vegetables and divide into three containers. Freeze two.

When you do your next vegetable mix prep, pull out your stock base and place on a low burner. As you prep, add scraps to your stock and simmer four hours adding water as needed, strain and refrigerate.

This is great also if you have vegetables that are on the verge of spoiling. Simply cut them Chunk-a Chunk-a and throw in. Other items you may or may not have thought of to use are:

Leaves and base head from celery
Outer pieces of onions, even the parts that are soft
or bruised
Potato peels

Tomato tops and bottoms
Tomato skins
Broccoli and cauliflower stems
Squash and zucchini peels, ends, and seeds with
    juice
Cucumber ends and peels
Swiss Chard stems
Any green leafy vegetable stems and outer leaves
Mushroom stems
Leftover vegetables (nothing with cheese or dairy)
Carrot tops, tips and peels
Root vegetable tops, tips and peels

Never putting herb in your stock, as each recipe calls for its own set of favors. Also avoid using hot peppers.

Condensed Soup Base

This base is for those times your recipe calls for a can of "Cream of _____ Condensed Soup". Using fresh ingredients from your garden or local farmer's market, as well as having complete control of ingredients due to your family's food allergies, will help you to get off the chemicals and over processed foods that may be causing weight gain and other health issues.

2 T butter OR vegetable oil
2 T vegetable stock
1 small onion & 2 cloves of garlic puréed OR 2 1/2 t onion powder & 1 t garlic powder
7 t A/P flour OR 3 1/2 t corn starch
1/8 t sea salt (optional)
1/8 t black pepper, coarsely ground
1 C whole milk, half & half, soy milk OR almond milk

1. In a heavy sauce pan, melt butter
2. Add vegetable stock and puréed mixture and stir for 30 seconds once it comes to a boil.
3. Whisk in flour, salt and pepper.
4. Simmer for one minute.
5. Add milk and stir constantly until mixture thickens.
6. Lower heat and cook for three minutes while stirring. Do not allow to scorch.
7. Remove from heat and allow to cool.
8. Continue with your recipe or place in an airtight container and refrigerate for no more than three days.

# Condiments and Sauces

## Relishes and Dressings

Catalina Dressing
Yield=2 C

2 H scallions, finely chopped
1/4 t black pepper, finely ground
1/2 t sea salt
1/4 C vinegar
1/2 C sugar, granulated
1/2 C tomato ketchup
1 C canola oil (do not use olive oil)

1. Place scallions, black pepper, sea salt in a mortar and pestle and process until scallions are almost paste.
2. Place in a bowl and add vinegar and sugar.
3. Beat until sugar is dissolved.
4. Stir in ketchup.

5. Whip dressing while slowly pouring in oil.
6. Incorporate well.
7. Refrigerate at least 24 hours before using.

## Garden Relish

1/2 head cauliflower, cut into flowerets
1 C All-American Trinity Mix, Chunk-a Chunk-a, 3/4 inch
1 1/2 C Mirepoix
1 4-oz jar slice pimiento
1/3 C green olives, pitted, drained
3/4 C vinegar
1/2 C extra virgin olive oil
2 T sugar
1 t sea salt
1/4 t black pepper, coarsely ground
1/2 t oregano leaves, dried
1/4 C water

1. Put all ingredients in a large pot and bring to a boil.
2. Simmer, covered, for five minutes. Do not over cook.
3. Cool to room temperature.
4. Place in a glass container and refrigerate at least 24 hours before serving, agitating the container every time you go to the refrigerator
5. Keep refrigerated for no longer than 3 months.

# Gravy

## Vegetable Gravy

1 H All-American Trinity Mix, finely chopped
1 C Vegetable Stock
1/2 T cornstarch dissolved in 2 T cold Vegetable
Stock

1. In a sauce pan, cook vegetable mix in stock until vegetables are tender, about 15 minutes.
2. Using a wire whip, stir broth while slowly adding cornstarch mixture.
3. Continue to cook for 8 minutes, stirring constantly.

## Summer Delight Frozen Dressing

1 C Raspberry OR Lime OR Orange OR Lemon Sherbet
4 T vinegar, white, rice, OR wine
4 t oregano
2 t garlic powder
1/2 t celery salt
6 fresh basil leaves, finely chopped
1 1/2 t black pepper, coarsely ground
1/2 t extra virgin olive oil
An ice tray or candy molds

1. Mix all ingredients except sherbet in a small bowl.
2. Without allowing the sherbet to melt, incorporate vinegar mixture into sherbet by pressing and folding.

3. Place in ice tray or molds, cover and place in freezer at least two hours.
4. When ready to use, place tray/molds in a shallow plate of hot water for 45-60 seconds and place one cube/molded piece in the center of the salad.
5. Allow dressing to melt slightly before serving.

Serving suggestion:
If you are having a hot summer's day luncheon, use ice trays and a couple of sherbet flavors, placing them in an insulated ice bucket with a lid and place on table. Serve with ice tongs.


## Tzatziki

2 cucumbers, peeled, seeded, coarsely chopped
1 T sea salt, finely ground
1 1/4 C Greek yoghurt
3 sprigs dill, stems removed
2 T olive oil
1 T lemon juice, freshly squeezed
2 1/2 t garlic, minced
1 t sea salt or to taste
1 1/2 t black pepper, coarsely ground

1. Place cucumbers in a strainer over a cold Vegetable Stockpot and mix with 1 T sea salt.
2. Allow to drain for 1 hour.
3. In a food processor or blender, place cucumbers and all remaining ingredients and mix thoroughly.
4. Place in a glass container, cover and refrigerate for 24 hours before serving.

# Mayonnaise-based Dressings

From cole slaw to chicken salad, these sauces and dressings will add the finishing touch on your dish. All recipes in this group are best made at least 24 hours before use.

<u>1000 Island Dressing</u>

1 C mayonnaise
1/4 C tomato ketchup
3 T sweet pickle relish
1/2 egg, hard boiled, finely chopped
1 H Cool Summer Mix, finely chopped

Mix all ingredients and refrigerate, covered, overnight.


<u>Cole Slaw Dressing</u>

1 C mayonnaise
1/4 C milk
2 T vinegar, apple cider
3 T sugar, superfine
2 t poppy seeds, whole
1 t celery salt
1 t black pepper, coarsely ground

1. Mix sugar and milk until sugar is dissolved.
2. Add rest of ingredients and mix until well incorporated.
3. Refrigerate.

## Russian Dressing

1 C mayonnaise
1/4 C tomato ketchup
2 or 3 drops hot sauce (optional)
1 t scallions, finely chopped

Blend all ingredients and refrigerate.


## Starch Salad Dressing

1 C mayonnaise
3 T vinegar
2 T yellow or spicy mustard
2 T milk
1 t celery salt
1 t garlic powder
1-2 drops hot sauce (optional)
2 t black pepper, finely ground
1 t sea salt, finely ground
1 hard boiled egg, finely chopped (optional)
1/4 C sweet pickle relish

Combine all ingredients and refrigerate.


## Tarter Sauce

1 C mayonnaise
1/4 C sweet pepper relish
1 drop hot sauce

Mix all ingredients and refrigerate.

## Fish & Meat Salad Dressing

This is the same as Starch Salad Dressing except you add 2 t lemon juice and 1 T Worcestershire Sauce.


## Quick Homemade Mayonnaise

1/4 C Egg Mix OR reconstituted powdered egg
1 T white vinegar
1 C canola, vegetable OR olive oil
P sea salt, finely ground
P garlic powder (optional)

1. In a bowl, whisk together egg and vinegar.
2. Continue to whip and slowly pour in oil in a steady stream.
3. Beat briskly until desired consistency.
4. Stir in salt to taste and garlic powder.
5. Refrigerate.

You can use a blender or mixer instead of doing this by hand, pouring oil while mixture is beating.

## Vinaigrette

1 T balsamic vinegar
2 t white wine vinegar
2 t brown mustard
3/4 t molasses
1/4 t honey
1 T sugar, superfine
1/2 t garlic powder
P sea salt
P black pepper, finely ground
6 T extra virgin olive oil

1. In a small bowl, mix together all ingredients except oil.
2. With a whisk, begin to beat mixture, adding oil, 1 T at a time.

# Sweet & Savory Sauces

## Butterscotch Sauce

1 C brown sugar, light, packed
1/4 C whipping cream
3 T unsalted butter
2 T Karo syrup, light

This should be made at least a half hour before serving

1. Combine all ingredients in a heavy saucepan.
2. Bring to a boil and cook for 3 minutes without stirring.
3. Remove from heat and let cool.

## Hot Fudge Sauce

3/4 C cocoa, unsweetened
6 T unsalted butter, melted
1 14-oz can sweetened condensed milk
1 t vanilla extract

1. In a small sauce pan over medium heat, beat together cocoa and butter with whisk.
2. Whip until smooth.
3. Add milk a little at a time, blending thoroughly between each addition.
4. Stir fudge using a wooden spoon until just about to simmer.
5. Remove from heat.
6. Stir in vanilla.
7. Use immediately or allow to cool.
8. Keep all leftovers refrigerated in a glass container with a tight fitting lid.

**Variations**
Add 1/4 t mint extract when you add the vanilla.
Add 1 P cinnamon with the cocoa.


## Light Tomato Sauce

**Note:** In the unabridged cookbook, this recipe uses a vegetable mix and a prep mix that is not included in this book.

1 C Vegetable Stock
1 C V-8 Juice
1 H All-American Trinity Mix, coarsely chopped
1 t fresh minced garlic
3 fresh mushrooms
3 slices zucchini, Coin Cut, 1/4 inch
3 basil leaves, finely chopped
1/2 t extra virgin olive oil
1 T cornstarch

1. Place All-American Trinity Mix, garlic, mushrooms and zucchini in a food processor and purée.
2. Mix 1/4 C V-8 Juice with cornstarch until completely dissolved. Set aside.
3. Place remaining V-8 juice and the rest of the unused ingredients in a sauce pan and bring to a simmer.
4. Simmer for 10 minutes.
5. Using a whisk, beat sauce while slowly pouring in cornstarch mixture.
6. Let simmer for 10 minutes stirring occasionally.

## Shrimp Cocktail Sauce

3:1 Ketchup : Prepared horseradish

Mix well and refrigerate for at least one hour. Will keep in refrigerator for up to two weeks.

# Spice Mixes

Apple Pie Spice Mix
4:2:1:1

Ground cinnamon
Ground nutmeg
Ground allspice
Ground cardamom

Mix thoroughly.

Pumpkin Pie Mix
4:2:1:1

Cinnamon, grated
Ginger, coarsely chopped
Cloves, whole
Nutmeg, grated

Place all in a mortar and work into a powder.

**Note:** You can also purchase ground versions of these spices and mix thoroughly, but make sure the spices are fresh when using. Open containers of spices lose their potency within 4 months or 6 months if refrigerated.

# Chapter 3: The Recipes

## Breakfast

### *Breakfast Twice-baked Potato*

1 white potato, baked, at room temperature
1 egg **OR** 4 ounces *Egg Mix*
1 T bacon, crumbled
1 T your favorite grated cheese
1 t parsley, finely chopped (optional)
Salt and pepper to taste

1. Lay potato on its side and cut off 1/2 inch from end-to-end. Throw small piece in your stock pot.
2. Sit potato upright, removing a little off the bottom, if needed, to make the potato sit flat.
3. Using a spoon, scoop out potato flesh, leaving 1/2 inch on the bottom and 1/4 inch on the sides. You now have a whole potato boat.
4. In a small bowl, mix together the potato flesh, bacon, cheese, parsley, salt and pepper.

5. Place the potato boat in a greased, oval au gratin dish.
6. Crack egg into the potato boat.
7. Bake in a 350°F oven for 6 minutes.
8. Remove from oven and cover potato and egg with potato flesh mixture.
9. Return to oven for four minutes or until cheese is bubbly.

## Variations

- Cover with *Light Tomato Sauce*.
- Add a finely chopped mushroom to cheese and potato flesh mixture.
- Serve with a dollop of sour cream.
- Smother with grilled onions.
- Top with Chili.
- Sauté *All-American Trinity Mix* and mix with potato flesh mixture.
- Use your imagination.

## *Burr Rarebit*

1/2 C Extra sharp cheddar cheese, grated or shredded
2 egg whites
2 egg yokes, beaten
1 t dry mustard
Splash Worcestershire sauce
2-3 drops hot sauce
P sea salt
P black pepper, coarsely ground
1 thick slice of bread (as if for Texas toast)

1. Toast the bread.
2. In a bowl, mix beaten egg yokes, mustard, cheese, Worcestershire sauce and hot sauce.
3. Beat egg whites to form stiff peaks.
4. Add a teaspoon of beaten egg whites to cheese mixture and stir.
5. Add sea salt and pepper.
6. Gently fold whites into cheese mixture, do not over mix, but try to keep the volume light and fluffy.
7. Place toast in a greased, shallow, oven-safe plate and top with egg mixture, covering toast completely.
8. Bake in a pre-heated 450°F oven for 10 minutes or until brown.

## *Morning snack/Pick-up Breakfast*

**Note:** This recipe will make four servings, however, it will keep up to two weeks in the refrigerator.

1 2.75-ounce package of flavored gelatin; lime, lemon or orange.
1 C boiling water
1 C ice-cold water
1 H fresh fruit (peaches, pears or mangoes are best), Chunk-a Chunk-a
3 T wheat germ, **OR** Grape-Nuts (not flakes), **OR** wheat germ w/honey
Plain or Vanilla yogurt **OR** cottage cheese

1. In a travel coffee mug or 10- to 14-ounce mug, place wheat germ in the bottom.
2. Top with fruit.
3. In a small bowl, dissolve gelatin in boiling water.
4. When completely dissolved, stir in ice-cold water.
5. Pour 1/2 C of gelatin in each mug and place in refrigerator until set.
6. Once the gelatin is set, top with 3/4 C yogurt or 2/3 C cottage cheese.
7. Cover with plastic wrap. If using travel mug, add the lid as well.
8. Set back into refrigerator.

To serve, grab them as you leave for work for a healthy mid-morning snack or grab one for breakfast on the go. Dig deep to the bottom and mix everything together before eating.

## *Vicki Quickie w/variations*

1 T Whole Hog Sausage, cooked, crumbled, drained
1 T Grated Cheddar Cheese
4 oz or 1/4 cup *Egg Mix*
1 *Biscuit Quickie* biscuit

1. On a flat iron griddle or small non-stick fry pan sprayed with pan release, pour in egg mix.
2. Cook slowly, busting bubbles if they form.
3. Once the egg starts to firm up, add sausage and cheese to the center of the egg.
4. Fold egg over to the center, rotating a quarter turn to form a small envelope full of sausage and egg. (pocket 1-egg omelet). Omelet should be the same size as your biscuit without much hangover.
5. Place pocket omelet inside biscuit.

## *Variations*

- Plain: Fold egg without adding any filling.
- Tom/Che: Replace sausage with coarsely chopped tomato.
- The Canadian: Use one slice of Canadian Bacon instead of Sausage.
- Winter Morning: Keep sandwich open and cover with sausage gravy.

# Soups

### Bean & Veggie Soup

2 H Great Northern Beans, Pinto Beans, **OR**
Cranberry Beans
P sea salt
Water
T olive oil
1 H *Cool Summer Mix*, coarsely chopped
1 H *Mirepoix*, Chunk-a Chunk-a
6 fresh basil leaves, snipped
1/4 t fresh garlic, minced
1/4 C fresh green beans
1/8 t black pepper, coarsely ground
2 C *Vegetable Stock*
1 H fresh spinach, turnip greens **OR** mustard greens,
finely chopped
1/4 C Buckwheat Groats

1. In a sauce pan, place beans and salt. Cover with 3 to 4 cups of water, insuring that water is at least 2 inches above the beans.
2. Cover and bring to a rolling boil.
3. Cook for 5 minutes.
4. Remove from heat and set aside, uncovered, for at least an hour.
5. In a crock pot, layer beans and remainder of ingredients in the order given, except for the groats.
6. Slow cook on high for 8-10 hours.
7. 30 minutes before serving, add groats, pressing them under the liquid.
8. Serve with assorted crackers.

## *Buttermilk Soup*

1 C buttermilk
3 H cucumbers, peeled finely chopped
2 H *Cool Summer Mix*, finely chopped
1/4 C half and half
1 1/2 t tarragon leaves, dried
1 1/2 t lemon juice, freshly squeezed
P sea salt
P black pepper, finely ground
Sour cream
Chives, snipped

1. Combine buttermilk, cucumbers, 1 H Cool Summer Mix, half and half, tarragon and lemon juice in a blender and purée.
2. Pour into a glass container and stir in 1 H Cool Summer Mix, salt and pepper.
3. Cover and chill for 12 hours.
4. Serve ice cold with a dollop of sour cream and chives.

# Condensed Cream Soups

### Condensed Cream of Celery Soup

3 C celery, finely chopped **OR** 3 C *Cool Summer Mix*, finely chopped
3 C *Vegetable Stock*
2 t fresh basil, finely chopped (optional)
1 *Condensed Soup Base* Prep Mix

1. Place celery and Vegetable Stock in a sauce pan and cook for 10 minutes, stirring occasionally.
2. Drain stock back into your stock pot.
3. Add basil.
4. Purée in blender or food processor.
5. Fold cooked puréed vegetables into *Condensed Soup Base* and stir over low heat for 1 minute.
6. Cover and refrigerate for no more than three days or continue with your recipe.

## Condensed Cream of Mushroom Soup

6 C mushrooms, finely chopped
4 C *Vegetable Stock*
1 t black pepper, coarsely ground
1 *Condensed Soup Base* Prep Mix

1. Place mushrooms and stock in a heavy sauce pan and cook for 10 minutes, stirring occasionally.
2. Drain the stock back into your stock pot.
3. Purée in blender or food processor.
4. Fold cooked, puréed mushrooms into Condensed Soup Base and stir over low heat for 1 minute.
5. Cover and refrigerate for no longer than three days or continue with your recipe.

## Homemade Creamed Soup

1. In a sauce pan over medium heat, add 1 C whole milk into prepared condensed vegetable soup and mix with a wire whip.
2. Heat thoroughly, but do not let boil.

## *Cool Fruit Soup*

1/2 C fruit, peeled, coarsely chopped **OR**
   1/2 C berries, washed, drained **OR**
   1/3 C melon, coarsely chopped
1/2 C plain or vanilla yogurt
1 t fresh lemon juice
2 T Vegetable Stock
1/4 t cinnamon **OR** ginger
1 T light rum **OR** Midori (optional)
Sprig of fresh mint for garnish (optional)

1. In a blender, purée all ingredients except mint, until smooth.
2. Place covered in refrigerator for at least 1 hour.
3. Serve in a chilled bowl and garnish with mint.

### Suggested Fruit

| | |
|---|---|
| Avocados | Peaches |
| Nectarines | Cantaloupe/Honeydew |
| Banana | Pears |
| Mango | Cherries |
| Blueberries | Seedless Blackberries |

### Cream of Sweet Potato Soup

1/2 C sweet potato, roasted, peeled, slightly warm
3/4 C *Vegetable Stock*
1 T *Mirepoix Mix*
2 t light brown sugar
1/8 t sea salt
1/8 t ground nutmeg or freshly grated
P black pepper, coarsely ground
1-2 drops hot sauce (optional)
2 T half and half
Dollop of sour cream (optional)

1. In a blender, purée sweet potato, Mirepoix, and stock.
2. In a sauce pan over medium heat, bring purée to a simmer.
3. Lower heat to medium-low.
4. Add next five ingredients and stir.
5. Cover and let simmer for 10 minutes.
6. Remove from heat and stir in half and half.
7. Refrigerate for at least 5 hours before serving in a chilled bowl.
8. Serve with a dollop of sour cream.

### *Vegetarian Onion Soup*

1 C *Vegetable Stock*
S Worcestershire sauce
3- to 4-inch of French bread, fresh or stale
3 H Spanish onion, Coin Cut, shaved
1 T olive oil
2-ounces 'Rice Vegan' mozzarella flavor, sliced

1. In an iron skillet, sauté onions in olive oil until onions are caramelized, adding Worcestershire sauce half way through.
2. In a 10-ounce French Onion Crock, place chunk of French bread.
3. Add onions, scraping skillet into the crock.
4. Fill with stock.
5. Top with vegan cheese, covering the entire opening of crock.
6. Broil four inches from heat source for 5-6 minutes or until cheese starts to brown.

# Salads

### Carrot Salad

2 H carrots, grated
1 T pineapple, crushed, with juice
1 T raisins, golden
1 t *Quick Homemade Mayonnaise*
1 cube *Summer Delight Frozen Dressing*

1. Mix first four ingredients and refrigerate, covered, for 1 hour.
2. Add frozen dressing cube 5 minutes before serving.

### *Creamy Cole Slaw*

1 C cabbage, shredded or grated
1/4 C carrots, grated
3 T red cabbage, grated
1/4 C *Tzatziki* (or more, if needed)

1. Combine all vegetables in a bowl.
2. Add Tzatziki.
3. Mix, adding more Tzatziki if needed to create a creamy slaw.
4. Refrigerate at least 1 hour.

**Note:** If you like, instead of adding more Tzatziki, add a cube of Summer Delight Frozen Dressing at serving time.

### Fruited Chicken Salad

1 H chicken breast, poached, chilled,
    Chunk-a Chunk-a
2 T *Golden Fruit Mix*
3 T *Cool Summer Mix*, finely chopped
3-oz scoop lemon sorbet, optional
2 H mesclun salad mix
1 T mayonnaise

1. In a small bowl, mix the first three ingredients.
2. Add mayonnaise and mix, adding more mayonnaise to taste.
3. Chill, covered, for at least 1 hour before serving.
4. Arrange salad mix on a salad plate and top with chicken salad.
5. Garnish with sorbet.

## Lunch Counter Salads

These salads may be used in sandwiches or on top of a *Two-Fisted Salad.*

### Tuna Salad
1 5-oz tuna, can or pouch, drained and separated with a fork.
2 H *All-American Trinity Mix*, coarsely chopped
1 T sweet pickle relish **OR** bread and butter pickles, coarsely chopped
1 t brown or spicy mustard
2 T *Quick Homemade Mayonnaise*

Mix all in a bowl and refrigerate for 1 hour.

### Ham Salad
1 H Deli Ham, coarsely chopped
2 H *All-American Trinity Mix*, finely chopped
1 T sweet pickle relish
1 t yellow **OR** brown mustard
1/2 hard boiled egg, coarsely chopped (optional)
2 T *Quick Homemade Mayonnaise*

Mix all ingredients, cover and refrigerate for one hour.

### Chicken Salad
1 H chicken, poached, Chunk-a Chunk-a
1 H *All-American Trinity Mix*, finely chopped
3/4 t sweet pickle relish
1 1/2 T *Quick Homemade Mayonnaise*

Mix all ingredients, cover and refrigerate for at least one hour.

### Shrimp Salad

1 H shrimp, mini, cooked (these usually are available in the frozen section of your grocery store and should be completely thawed before use)
1 H *Cool Summer Mix*
1/2 t lemon juice
1/2 t *Shrimp Cocktail Sauce*
1 T *Quick Homemade Mayonnaise*

Mix all ingredients, cover and refrigerate for at least one hour.

**Note:** Please remember to refrigerate all dishes made with mayonnaise.

### Summer Delight Salad

3H Mixed salad greens
1H *Cool Summer Mix*, coarsely chopped
1oz Gouda Cheese
1oz Monterey Jack and/or Pepper Jack Cheese, cut in strips
1oz Swiss Cheese, cut in strips
1oz American Cheese, cut in strips
2 prunes, stewed, chilled (optional)
2 T *Garden Relish*
1/4 C cottage cheese
1/4 C yoghurt, vanilla
1/2 C berries (in season or frozen, thawed)
1/2 C fruit, sliced (in season; frozen, thawed; canned, drained)
1 deviled egg OR 1 pickled egg, sliced
1 molded *Summer Delight Frozen Dressing*

1. Toss together greens and Cool Summer Mix and place in serving plate.
2. Arrange rest of ingredients creatively on top of lettuce mixture, placing the un-molded dressing in the middle.
3. Allow five minutes to let the dressing melt just a tad.

**Note:** The original Summer Delight (cir 1975) did not have the frozen dressing, but instead had three 1oz scoops of sherbet: 1 scoop of orange, 1 scoop of lime and 1 scoop of lemon. It also did not have the yoghurt nor berries and the prunes were not optional. The salad was served with Catalina Dressing. Over the years, I modified this 'Summer Menu Only' salad to what it is today.

## *Two-Fisted Salad with Variations*

1 H mixed salad greens **OR** Musclun Mix
1 H *Mirepoix Mix*, Chunk-a Chunk-a
1 cube or mold *Summer Delight Frozen Dressing*, any flavor

Mix greens with Mirepoix Mix and top with dressing cube.

## Variations

- Add another handful of greens for a 3-fisted salad
- Add 1/4 C Garden Relish
- Add a hard-boiled egg, sliced and another handful of greens for a lunch entrée.

# Sides

### *Asparagus Casserole*

1 H asparagus, whole, steamed
1 hard boiled egg, sliced
1/2 C grated cheese
1/3 C *Condensed Cream of Celery Soup*

1. In a 10-ounce au gratin dish, layer in this order:
   - Asparagus
   - Egg
   - 1/4 C cheese
   - Condensed soup
   - Rest of cheese
2. Bake in pre-heated 350°F oven for 20 minutes.
3. Serve with optional hot sauce and sour cream

### Broccoli Casserole

5 T minute rice
1 H broccoli florets
1 H *Cool Summer Mix*, coarsely chopped
1 T butter, unsalted
5 T cold water
3 T *Condensed Cream of Mushroom Soup*
1/2 C sharp cheddar cheese, shredded
2 T bread crumbs
1 H broccoli or alfalfa sprouts

1. In a bowl, mix first 7 ingredients.
2. Place in a greased 10 or 14 ounce soufflé cup.
3. Cover with foil and place in a 350°F oven for 18 minutes.
4. Uncover cup and sprinkle on bread crumbs.
5. Return to oven and bake uncovered for 12 minutes or until bread crumbs are a golden brown.
6. Garnish with sprouts.

### Variations

- Substitute cauliflower for broccoli.
- Substitute broccoflower for broccoli.

## *Buckwheat Groats Pilaf*

1/2 C *Vegetable Stock*
1/4 C Buckwheat groats
P sea salt, optional
1 H *All-American Trinity Mix*, finely chopped
1 T olive oil

1. In a small, heavy, oven-safe sauce pan with a tight fitting lid, sauté All-American Trinity Mix in olive oil until onions are translucent.
2. Add Vegetable Stock and salt.
3. Bring to a full, rolling boil.
4. Add groats and stir until mixture returns to a full boil.
5. Cover and place in a pre-heated 350°F oven for 18 minutes.
6. Remove from oven and let sit covered for 5 minutes.
7. Remove lid, stir and serve.

### Carrot Casserole

4 T carrots, cooked, mashed
1 T butter, unsalted
P cinnamon
1 1/2 T *Egg Mix*
2 T sugar
3/4 T *Self-rising Flour*

1. Place all ingredients in a blender and blend well.
2. Pour mixture into a greased 8-oz soufflé cup
3. Place cup in a shallow pan and place on oven rack.
4. Fill pan with hot water, being careful not to allow any water to go inside the cup.
5. Bake in pre-heated 350°F oven for 35 to 45 minutes; until inserted knife comes out clean.

### *Daddy's Cucumbers*

1/2 medium-sized cucumber, peeled, coin cut 1/4 inch.
2 T white vinegar OR juice from a jar of pickle
1 t sea salt
P black pepper, coarsely ground or to taste
4 or 5 large ice cubes

1. Dissolve salt in vinegar.
2. Placed sliced cucumbers into a serving bowl and pour vinegar over top.
3. Add pepper and mix.
4. Top with ice cubes and let sit at room temperature for 20 minutes before serving.

*Variation:* Add a slice of sweet onion, coin cut, shaved.

**Note:** You can use the leftover liquid to do another batch.

### *Refrigerator Pickles*

4 C cucumbers, coin cut, regular
1 T sea salt
1/2 C vinegar, white
1 medium onion, coin cut, shaved
2 t celery seed
1 C sugar

1. In a saucepan, heat salt, vinegar, celery seed and sugar until sugar is dissolved.
2. Remove from heat and let cool.
3. In a pint jar, layer cucumbers, then onions.
4. Pour in cooled vinegar mixture.
5. Screw on lid and shake jar.
6. Place in refrigerator for 48 hours, shaking the jar every time you go to the refrigerator.

**Note:** Make sure you keep this pickle refrigerated.

### *Spaghetti Squash with Tomato Sauce*

1 small spaghetti squash
*Vegetable Stock*
3/4 C *Light Tomato Sauce*
P black pepper, coarsely ground
Parmesan or Romano Cheese, grated

1. Cut squash in half and scoop out seeds.
2. Place squash, cut side down, in a baking pan.
3. Pour 1/4 inch of vegetable stock.
4. Roast in pre-heated 350°F oven for 40 minutes or until tender.
5. Heat tomato sauce.
6. Hold spaghetti squash with Tea towel and using a dinner fork, scrape meat onto serving plate.
7. Top with tomato sauce, cheese and offer freshly ground pepper to guests.

### Texas Vegetables

2 T Lentils, dry, washed
Boiling water
P sea salt
5 T *Mirepoix*, finely chopped
2 T tomatoes, finely chopped
3 T commercial BBQ Sauce
1-2 drops of hot sauce

1. Place Lentils in a bowl and pour boiling water to 1 inch above lentils. Add salt and cover for 2 hours.
2. In a sauce pan, add all ingredients including lentils and water.
3. Simmer for 1 1/2 hours or until lentils are tender, stirring occasionally.

## Variations

- Double lentils and serve on a warmed taco topped with shredded lettuce.
- Place 2 T refried beans on a warmed taco. Add Texas Veggies and top with shredded lettuce and grated cheese.
- Place 2 T cooked chicken or beef in a warmed taco or hamburger bun. Top with Texas Veggies and top with shredded lettuce and grated cheese.

## *Twice Baked Sweet Potatoes*

Sweet potatoes have very thin skins. I have found that if you bake the sweet potato to where the outer is done, but the center needs to bake a little longer is best used for this recipe. Make sure the potato is cool or at room temperature when making this dish.

1 medium size sweet potato, baked, halved
1 H *Cool Summer Mix*, finely chopped
1/4 t extra virgin oil
2 T cream cheese
1 T mozzarella cheese, shredded
P cinnamon
1/2 t butter
Crumbled bacon for garnish, optional

1.  Scoop out sweet potato, leaving at least 1/4-inch on all sides.
2.  Sauté *Cool Summer Mix* in olive oil using an iron skillet.
3.  Mix potato with all remaining ingredients except bacon.
4.  Place mixture into potato shell and top with bacon.
5.  Bake in pre-heated 350°F oven for 30 minutes **OR** microwave at 70% for 1.5 minutes, turning once.

# Entrées

## *Beef 'n Burger*

4 oz lean ground beef
1 H *All-American Trinity Mix*, coarsely chopped
1 t fresh garlic, minced
1/2 bay leaf
1/4 t dried oregano leaves
4 cherry tomatoes, sliced in half
1/4 t black pepper, coarsely ground
1 t white vinegar
1 t tomato paste
A few drops of hot sauce, to taste
1 T olive oil
1 Whole Wheat hamburger roll

1. Pour olive oil into skillet on medium heat.
2. Add All-American Trinity Mix, garlic, bay leaf and oregano.
3. Stir and let cook for 5 minutes.
4. Crumble ground beef into skillet and simmer until beef is well done.
5. Add cherry tomatoes, black pepper, vinegar and tomato paste.
6. Stir and let simmer on low for 20 minutes, stirring occasionally.
7. Remove bay leaf and stir in hot sauce.
8. Spoon onto hamburger roll.

### Variations
- Add 1 t unsweetened cocoa when you add the cherry tomatoes.

- Spoon mixture over 1/2 C cooked pasta. Do not use roll.
- Serve over *Buckwheat Groats Pilaf*. Do not use roll.
- Serve with *Creamy Cole Slaw*.

## *Coast to Coast Meatloaf*

This recipe was created in the 80's when I owned Coast to Coast Catering and Carry-out in Key West, Florida. The idea was to provide a 'leftover-style' meatloaf in which sandwiches were made the following day. I did a lot of thinking about whether to size it down or present it in its original form. I decided on the latter.

The recipe makes a 9-inch loaf of meatloaf. Each serving is a 1-inch slice and is great served hot or cold on a sub roll, onion roll, toasted bread or Cuban bread with all the trimmings. It freezes great as well.

1 1/2 lb. ground beef, 80-90% lean
1/2 lb. ground lamb
1 1/2 C *Cool Summer Mix*, finely chopped
1/4 C *Egg Mix*
1/4 C milk
1/2 C oatmeal, steel cut
3/4 C 'KC Masterpiece BBQ Sauce' (original) **OR** your favorite BBQ sauce
1 T oregano leaves, dried
2 T parsley, fresh, finely chopped
2 t table salt
2 T black pepper, coarsely ground
5 cloves garlic, whole
2 H cheddar cheese, 1/2-inch cubes
3 hard boiled eggs, peeled, whole
2 sprigs rosemary
Extra BBQ sauce

1. In a bowl, mix the first 11 ingredients.
2. Shape into loaf and place in a 9-inch loaf pan.

3. Make five holes with your finger, evenly spaced, in meatloaf and insert garlic. Close holes.
4. Make three holes and do the same thing with the hard boiled eggs.
5. Press cheese cubes into meatloaf in varying depths covering each one with meat.
6. Smooth top of meatloaf with your hand.
7. Pour a 1-inch wide strip lengthwise of BBQ Sauce.
8. Place sprigs of Rosemary on top of BBQ Sauce.
9. Place in a pre-heated 375°F for 10 minutes.
10. Reduce oven temperature to 350°F for 45 minutes.
11. Remove from oven and drain the juices.
12. Let set in the pan for 30 minutes.
13. Turn meatloaf out onto a sheet of foil and wrap tightly.
14. Refrigerate for 24 hours.
15. Remove and discard rosemary sprigs before slicing.

## Crab Alfredo

This recipe uses imported Parmigiano-Reggiano Cheese. Do not use anything else, otherwise it will not turn out creamy and what you will end up with will be a fine mess.

1 serving of fettuccine
1/4 C backfin crab (do not break lumps)
2 T butter, salted, softened
3 oz Parmigiano-Reggiano Cheese, freshly grated
2 t parsley, finely chopped

1. In a 2-quart pot, bring 1 1/2 quarts of water to a boil.
2. Place a strainer on top of the pot with your crab meat in it.
3. Add fettuccine and cook according to package instructions.
4. While pasta is cooking and crab meat is heating, beat together cheese and butter until creamy.
5. Place sauce in a large bowl.
6. When pasta is done, strain, leaving a small amount of water in the pasta and place in bowl with sauce.
7. Add crab and toss. You can use two methods of tossing. Either use tongs to lift pasta up and down until all ingredients are mixed, or use the 'panning for gold' method. This method is where you toss everything up and catch it in mid-air (it is all in the wrist).
8. Place on serving plate and sprinkle with parsley.

## *Variations*

- Replace crab with a handful of steamed, peeled shrimp.
- Replace crab with 3 ounces of poached chicken breast, Chunk-a Chunk-a.
- Replace crab with 1 T roasted sunflower seeds <u>and</u> 1 T shelled pistachio nuts.

## Curry Chicken & Fruit Salad

This is great for Brunch, Lunch or a light Supper.

1/2 C chicken breast, skinned, poached,
    Chunk-a Chunk-a
1 H *Cool Summer Mix*, coarsely chopped
1 H *Golden Fruit Mix*
1 T pecans, toasted, finely chopped
1/8 t black pepper, coarsely ground
1/8 t curry powder
1 1/2 T *Quick Homemade Mayonnaise*
2 H shredded lettuce

1. Mix all ingredients, except lettuce, in a bowl.
2. Cover and refrigerate for at least one hour.
3. Serve over lettuce.

### Devilish Crab Coins

4 ounces backfin crab
1/4 C bread crumbs
1/4 C *Egg Mix*
1/4 t Old Bay Seasoning
1/2 t Worcestershire sauce
1 T *Quick Homemade Mayonnaise*
1/4 t brown mustard
2 T vegetable oil **OR** peanut oil

1. In a bowl, combine egg mix, Old Bay, Worcestershire sauce, mayonnaise and mustard.
2. Gently add crabmeat and mix without breaking the lumps of crab.
3. Add bread crumbs.
4. Shape into 2-inch balls and place on a wax paper-lined cookie sheet, flattening each one with the bottom of a glass.
5. Cover and refrigerate at least one hour.
6. In an iron skillet, heat oil.
7. Fry crab coins for 5 minutes on each side or until golden brown.
8. Place fried crab coins on a paper towel, then transfer to dinner plate.
9. Serve with your favorite sauces.

This recipe will also make one nice crab cake, perfect to serve on a toasted, whole grain roll with all the trimmings.

### *Fruited Pork Chops w/Roasted Red Potatoes*

1 lean pork chop, 1 1/2-inch thick, butterflied
1 H *Savory Dried Fruit Mix*
1 H small red potatoes, scrubbed (do not peel)
1 t rosemary leaves, snipped
P black pepper, coarsely ground
P sea salt

1. Place fruit mix on one side of butterflied pork chop and close, securing chop with a toothpick.
2. Place in a round au gratin dish that has been greased with olive oil.
3. Sprinkle chop with rosemary leaves, pepper and salt.
4. Surround chop with potatoes.
5. Bake in a pre-heated 350°F oven for 30 minutes or until the internal temperature of the pork chop reaches 170°F.

### *Hoppin' John w/Sun Dried Tomatoes*

2 H black-eyed peas, cooked
1 C *Vegetable Stock*
1/2 C long grain rice
2 T extra virgin olive oil
2 T *Cool Summer Mix,* finely chopped
3 sun-dried tomatoes, Chunk-a Chunk-a
Sea salt
Black pepper, coarsely ground

1.  In a small iron skillet, sauté Cool Summer Mix in 2 t olive oil until onions are slightly soft.
2.  Transfer into an oven-safe sauce pan with a tight-fitting lid.
3.  Add remaining oil, peas, and stock.
4.  Stir and bring to a simmer, stirring occasionally.
5.  Pour in rice and bring to a rapid boil while stirring constantly.
6.  Remove from heat, add tomatoes on top and cover.
7.  Immediately place in a pre-heated 350°F oven for 18-20 minutes, or until all liquid has been absorbed.
8.  Salt and pepper to taste.

## *Lamb & Mushroom Pie*

4 ounces lamb, rib roast, Chunk-a Chunk-a
2 H mushrooms, coin cut, thin
1 H cherry tomatoes, smashed
1 H *Mirepoix,* finely chopped
1 T olive oil
1/2 t black pepper, coarsely ground
1/4 t sea salt, finely ground
1/4 t rosemary leaves, finely chopped
1/3 C *Vegetable Stock*
1 T corn starch
1 full recipe *Biscuit Quickie*, divided

1. In an iron skillet, cook lamb, vegetables and olive oil, browning lamb on all sides.
2. Add salt, rosemary and Vegetable Stock and let simmer for 10 minutes.
3. Remove 5 T of broth and mix with cornstarch until dissolved.
4. While stirring lamb and vegetables, slowly pour in cornstarch mixture, avoiding lumps to form.
5. Cook 5 minutes, stirring occasionally to prevent scorching.
6. Remove from heat.
7. Press 1/2 of the Biscuit Quickie dough into the bottom of a 10-ounce soufflé cup, allowing dough to go up the edges.
8. Roll the other half of dough into a ball and flatten with the palm of your hand.
9. Pour skillet contents into pastry lined cup and top with flattened dough.
10. Using a dinner fork, prick holes in top dough for venting.
11. Bake in a pre-heated 350°F oven for 15-20 minutes or until crust is golden brown.

## *Roasted Brussels Sprout and Carrot Pie*

1 H Brussels sprouts, quartered
1 H baby carrots, whole
1 H *Cool Summer Mix*, coarsely chopped
2 T olive oil
1/3 C *Mushroom Condensed Soup*
1/3 C Vegetable Stock
P thyme, dry
P oregano, dry
1 *Biscuit Quickie* recipe

1. Cut biscuit dough in half and roll each half out on a floured surface.
2. Place one rolled biscuit dough in a 10-ounce au gratin dish and press to cover the bottom and sides.
3. Coat Brussels sprouts, baby carrots and Cool Summer Mix in olive oil.
4. Place in a single layer on a heavy sheet pan that has been sprayed generously with pan release.
5. Roast veggies in a 450°F oven for 30 minutes, turning veggies after 15 minutes.
6. Place condensed soup, broth, thyme and oregano into a sauce pan and heat on low, stirring occasionally but do not let boil.
7. Place roasted veggies into soup mixture and stir.
8. Place mixture into prepared 10-ounce au gratin dish and top with rolled biscuit dough trimming any extra dough.
9. Using a sharp knife, cut out a small quarter-inch hole in dough for ventilation.
10. Bake in a 375°F oven for 30 minutes or until biscuit topping is golden brown.

### *Summer Lemonade Tuna*

1 3/4-inch fresh tuna steak
2 T frozen lemonade concentrate
2 t black pepper, coarsely ground
1 t sea salt
5 Lemon basil leaves, fresh (optional)
1 T vegetable oil or olive oil
2 slices fresh lemon, coin cut, regular

1.  Whisk together concentrate, pepper, salt and oil.
2.  Place tuna steak in an au gratin dish and pour liquid over.
3.  Put in refrigerator for 3 minutes.
4.  Add basil and place 4 inches below a heated broiler.
5.  After 5 minutes, turn tuna over and spoon juices over tuna steak.
6.  Top tuna with lemon slices.
7.  Continue to broil, about 3-5 minutes longer until internal temperature reaches 125°F.
8.  Do not over cook.

**Note:** Try some fresh thyme or finely chopped parsley, if you do not have lemon basil.

### *Swiss Hammer*

1 whole grain hamburger roll or kaiser roll, toasted
3 ounces thin-sliced deli ham
2 T your favorite BBQ sauce
1 slice Swiss cheese
Dill pickle wedge

1. In a small bowl, mix ham and BBQ sauce.
2. Microwave mixture on high for 60 seconds.
3. Stir and top with cheese.
4. Microwave on high for 45 seconds or until cheese is bubbly.
5. Carefully tilt bowl and slide ham mixture neatly onto toasted bun.
6. Garnish with pickle.

This is great with *Creamy Cole Slaw*, on the sandwich, or on the side!

# Breads

## *Baked Soup and Snack Crackers*

1 *Pie Pastry Recipe*
Sea salt
Assorted herbs, coarsely ground

1. Cut dough in half.
2. Roll dough as thin as you can (1/8-inch or less), on a floured surface.
3. Using a floured knife or cookie cutter, cut into 1- to 2-inch squares.
4. Place squares on an un-greased cookie sheet.
5. Using a fork, prick holes into each cracker.
6. Sprinkle with sea salt and/or herbs for different flavors.
7. Bake in a 400°F oven for 10 minutes or until golden brown.
8. Store in an air-tight container or bag.

## *Variations*
- When making your pie dough, use Whole Wheat flour option.
- Sprinkle 4:1 sugar:cinnamon in place of the salt and herbs.

### Biscuit Quickie

1/3 C *Self-rising Flour*
2 T plus 2 t milk
1 T *Quick Homemade Mayonnaise*

1. Preheat oven to 400°F.
2. Mix all ingredients until just blended, do not over mix.
3. Drop from spoon onto lightly greased baking sheet.
4. Bake 12 minutes or until golden brown.

YIELD=2 biscuits

## *Hint of Honey Soda Bread*

Great served with soup and stews!

2 C whole wheat flour
1 t table salt
1 t baking soda
2 T honey
1 C buttermilk **OR** 3/4 C apple sauce plus 1/4 C apple juice
1 egg, slightly beaten

1. In a large mixing bowl, combine flour, salt and baking soda.
2. Make a well in the center of flour mixture and add honey, buttermilk and egg.
3. Stir until slightly moistened. Batter will be soft.
4. Pour in a greased, 1-qt casserole dish.
5. Bake in a pre-heated 375°F oven for 20-25 minutes.
6. Cool completely before slicing.

## *Holiday Pumpkin Muffins*

This muffin batter MUST be made at least 24 hours in advance. It will thicken to the correct consistency when placed covered in the refrigerator. This recipe will yield two loaves or 3-dozen muffins. I personally make just muffins, making just the number I need. They are at the peak of their flavor right out of the oven. The batter will keep up to three weeks, however, I usually divide the batch in half and give one half to a friend. Makes a great gift!

3 C sugar, granulated
1 C vegetable oil
1 C *Egg Mix*
1 15-ounce canned pumpkin (do not use pumpkin pie mix)
3 1/2 C A/P flour
2 t baking soda
1 t salt
1 t baking powder
1 T *Pumpkin Pie Spice*
1/2 t cloves
2/3 C water

1. In a large bowl, mix sugar and oil.
2. Add pumpkin and Egg Mix.
3. Beat well.
4. Sift in flour, baking soda, salt, baking powder and spices.
5. Mix until incorporated.
6. Add water and beat by hand for 2 minutes.
7. Let set overnight in an air-tight container in the refrigerator.

*Muffins*

1. Grease muffin tin or 8-ounce soufflé cup.
2. Fill 2/3 full.
3. Bake in a pre-heated 350°F oven for 14-18 minutes or until muffins are lightly brown and an inserted toothpick comes out clean.

*Loaf*

1. Grease loaf pan.
2. Pour half the batter and smooth with spatula.
3. Bake in the center of a pre-heated 325°F oven for 1 1/2 hours or until golden brown and inserted knife comes out clean.

# Desserts

## *All-American Fruit Pies*

Each of these recipes are classic fruit pies. If you have made and rolled out your dough ahead of time, these are very easy and quick to do. Each of these fruit pie recipes will make six 10-oz soufflé cups **OR** a 9-inch pie. If you use the soufflé cups, the bottom pastry is optional.

### *Apple Pie*

6 C Granny Smith apples, peeled, cored, half moon,
    regular
1 1/2 t apple pie spice
3/4 C sugar
2 T tapioca
1 T butter, unsalted, cut into 6 pieces
Egg Wash
Pie pastry for six 10-oz soufflé cups

1. In a large bowl, toss together apples, sugar, spices and tapioca.
2. Let sit for 15 minutes.
3. Place apple mixture evenly in pastry-lined soufflé cups (pastry optional)
4. Place one piece of butter on each cup.
5. Place top pastry, sealing edges. If you did not cut out a vent hole in your top pastry, make a slit in the top for venting.
6. Brush on Egg Wash.
7. Place pies in a pre-heated 400°F oven for 40 minutes or until bubbly and crust is golden brown.
8. Serve warm, room temperature or cold.

### Blackberry Pie

5 C blackberries, washed, drained
1 C sugar
1/4 C tapioca
1 T butter, cut into 6 pieces
Egg wash
Pie pastry

Instructions are same as for Apple Pie.

### Blueberry Pie

Same as Blackberry Pie, substituting blueberries for blackberries and adding 1 T lemon juice.

### Cherry Pie

Same as Blackberry Pie, substituting cherries, fresh, pitted for blackberries and adding an additional 1/4 C sugar.

### *Golden Fruit Pie*

6 C Golden Fruit Mix
1 t cinnamon, ground
1/2 t nutmeg, freshly grated
Juice from 1 lemon, strained
3/4 C light brown sugar
1/4 C honey
3 T tapioca
1 T unsalted butter, cut into 6 pieces
Egg Wash
Pie pastry

Glaze
1 T unsalted butter, melted
1/2 C milk (do not use skim)
Powdered sugar
1/2 t vanilla extract (use clear vanilla if you have it)

1. In a large bowl, toss together fruit, sugar, honey, spices and tapioca.
2. Let sit for 15 minutes.
3. Place fruit mixture evenly in six 10-oz soufflé cups, pastry-lined
4. Place one piece of butter on each cup.
5. Place top pastry, sealing edges. If you did not cut out a vent hole in your top pastry, make a slit in the top for venting.
6. Place in pre-heated 375°F oven for 40 minutes or until bubbly and crust is golden brown.
7. Cool pies on wire racks.
8. To make the glaze, in a small bowl, whip together milk and butter.
9. Slowly add sugar a little at a time until it resembles Elmer's Glue.
10. Stir in vanilla extract.

11. Drizzle glaze on cool pies and allow glaze to firm up
12. Serve pies at room temperature.
13. Refrigerate leftovers.

### *Pineapple Pie*

2 1/2 C crushed pineapple, drained, reserve juice (do
not use canned packed in syrup)
2 T cornstarch
1/2 C sugar
1/4 t salt
1 T butter, unsalted
1 T lemon juice
Pie Pastry

1. Place crushed pineapple, 2 T juice, sugar, and salt
   in a heavy saucepan over medium heat.
2. Mix cornstarch in remaining juice until cornstarch
   is dissolved.
3. Once mixture is about to boil, briskly stir in
   cornstarch mixture.
4. Stir until it begins to thicken.
5. Remove from heat and add lemon juice, stir.
6. Pour into to 8-oz or 10-oz soufflé cups lined with
   pastry.
7. Dot each cup with butter.
8. Place top pastry, sealing edges. If you did not cut
   out a vent hole in your top pastry, make a slit in
   the top for venting.
9. Bake in a pre-heated 350°F oven for 40 minutes or
   until crust is golden brown.
10. Serve at room temperature or chilled.

### *Red Pear & Cherry Pie*

Same as Blackberry Pie, substituting 4 C red pears,
peeled, cored, Half Moon, regular and 1 C fresh
cherries, washed and pitted.

## Creamery Muffin

1/3 C *Self-rising Flour*
1/3 C Vanilla ice cream, softened (or any other flavor)

1. Grease an 8-ounce soufflé cup.
2. Mix both ingredients and put into prepared cup.
3. Bake in a pre-heated 425°F oven for 10 minutes or until inserted toothpick comes out clean.
4. Cool in cup for 10 minutes before removing to cool completely or to serve.

**REMEMBER** it is only as sinful as the ice cream flavor you use.

### Peach Betty with variations

1/2 C peaches, fresh, Chunk-a Chunk-a
1/4 C brown sugar, light
1/4 C A/P flour
P nutmeg
P cinnamon
2 T butter, softened

1. Place peaches in a greased 10-ounce soufflé cup.
2. In a small bowl, mix sugar, flour and spices.
3. Cut in butter until mixture is crumbly.
4. Sprinkle flour mixture over peaches.
5. Bake in a microwave at 50% for 2 minutes. Turn and bake for 1 minute at 100% or until warm and bubbly.

Serving suggestion: Serve warm with Clotted Cream or your favorite ice cream.

### Variations

- Replace peaches with apples for an Apple Betty.
- Replace peaches with blueberries for a Blueberry Betty.
- Replace peaches with mango for a Mango Betty.
- Replace peaches with bananas. Top with vanilla ice cream and *Hot Fudge Sauce* for a Banana Betty with an Attitude.

## *Poached Pear w/Butterscotch Sauce*

1 1/2 C cranberry-apple juice cocktail
1 Bosc pear, peeled with stem intact
1/4 C Simple Syrup
P Apple Pie Spice
Butterscotch Sauce

1.  In a small skillet or shallow sauce pan, mix juice, simple syrup and spices.
2.  Bring to a simmer.
3.  Add pear and poach, turning and basting frequently.
4.  Poach until pear is tender and has taken on a light pink color.
5.  To serve, place poached pear in a round au gratin dish, stem side up, and pour warm Butterscotch Sauce over the pear. Garnish with mint leaf.

**Note:** Leftover sauce can be refrigerated and heated in the microwave.

### Quick Fix Pudding

1T sugar, granulated
1/4 t brown sugar, light
1 3/4 t cornstarch
P salt, table
1/2 C milk, whole
1/4 t vanilla extract

1. Mix sugars, cornstarch and salt in a saucepan.
2. Add milk and cook over medium heat, stirring constantly.
3. When mixture thickens, add vanilla and continue to stir and cook for 3 minutes.
4. Pour into soufflé cups and chill for 4 hours OR continue with your recipe.

**Note:** For chocolate pudding, melt 10 chocolate chips in the microwave. Pour melted chocolate into pudding when you add the vanilla. For butterscotch pudding, use butterscotch chips.

### *Seven-day Cobbler*

This dish was created to offer variety during the week. Use at least three kinds of fresh fruit. This keeps well, if covered, in the refrigerator. Serve warm by placing covered, but vented, in the microwave for 30-40 seconds. The recipe makes 7 cobblers made in 8-ounce soufflé cups.

Fruit
Apples, Peaches, or Pears: 1/2 C
Blackberries, Blueberries, or Raspberries: 3/4 C

*Fruit Preparation*

For apple, peach and pear: peel, core and cut 1/4-inch half moon.
For berries: wash and drain well.

1. Place fruit in the bottom of 7 well greased soufflé cups.
2. Sprinkle each with 1 1/2 t sugar, granulated or superfine.
3. Sprinkle a P of Apple Pie Spice on apple if desired.
4. Let set for 10 minutes.
5. Meanwhile, make batter.

*Batter*

1 egg
3/4 C sugar, granulated
1/4 C milk, whole
1 C A/P flour

1 t baking powder
1/2 t table salt
1/2 t vanilla extract
2 T butter, unsalted, melted

1. Beat together egg, sugar and milk.
2. Sift together flour, baking powder and salt into egg mixture and stir until well incorporated.
3. Stir in vanilla extract.
4. Pour in melted butter and blend well.
5. Divide batter between prepared soufflé cups, insuring that all fruit is covered and batter touches the sides of the cups.
6. Bake in a pre-heated 350°F oven for 30 minutes.
7. Let cool for 15-20 minutes before serving.

## *Topsy Turvy Cake with Variations*

1/2 C Yellow Cake Mix, complete
2 T Water

1. Beat water and cake mix until smooth. If batter is too stiff, add more water 1/4 t at a time.
2. Pour into greased 7-or 8-oz soufflé cup.
3. Microwave on high for 1 minute.
4. Turn.
5. Continue to microwave on high for 30-45 seconds until inserted toothpick comes out clean.
6. Let cool in cup for 5 minutes.
7. Run a knife around edge of cake.
8. Invert onto serving dish.

**Note:** For a 9-inch square cake, use 2 C mix to 1/2 C water.

## Variations

### *Traditional Pineapple Topsy Turvy Cake*
Place 2 T brown sugar and 2 t butter in greased 10oz soufflé cup. Microwave for 30-45 seconds or until liquid. Add 2 T pineapple tidbits, drained, reserve juice and a maraschino cherry. Use juice to make batter and continue with recipe.

### *Sometimes you feel like a nut ...*
In your greased soufflé cup, place a 4-inch piece of your favorite candy bar or a chocolate-covered cherry. Continue with recipe.

### Fruit Topsy Turvy Cake

Mix 1/4 C of fresh fruit or berry with 1 t *Simple Syrup* and let sit for 5 minutes. Pour into greased soufflé cup and continue.

### Butterscotch Coconut

Place 2oz **Butterscotch Sauce** in greased soufflé cup. Sprinkle in 2T shredded coconut. Continue with recipe.

### Chocolate Fudge Topsy Turvy Cake

Add 1t unsweetened cocoa to cake mix. In greased soufflé cup, place 1H chocolate chips and melt slightly. Continue with recipe.

### Nutty Topsy Turvy Cake

9 pieces of walnuts, black walnuts, OR pecans. You may use them either whole or coarsely chopped. Mix with 3T King Syrup OR treacle. Place mixture in greased soufflé cup. Continue with recipe. You can also add 1 t coconut to this for something different.

### Apple Spice Topsy Turvy Cake

Mix 1 t *Apple Pie Spice* and 1/2 t cinnamon into cake mix. Place 1/8 C chunky applesauce into bottom of greased soufflé cup. Continue with recipe.

### Chocolate Marble Topsy Turvy Cake

Make a double batch of batter. Melt 6 chocolate chips and blend with 1T of batter. Place 2oz Hot Fudge Sauce in a greased 10oz soufflé cup. Pour in plain batter. Place chocolate batter in center and swirl with a sharp knife point. Continue with recipe.

## USE YOUR IMAGINATION FOR EVEN BETTER TREATS!

## *Whole Wheat Sugar Cookies*

1 C sugar, granulated
1 t baking powder
1/2 t salt
1/2 t baking soda
1/2 C butter-flavored shortening
2 T milk
1 t apple pie spice
1 t vanilla extract
1/4 C *Egg Mix*
2 C whole wheat flour

<u>Topping</u>
2 t sugar, granulated
1/2 t cinnamon, ground
1/2 pound M&M's (optional)
Pecans (optional)

1. Preheat oven to 375°F.
2. In large bowl, combine first 10 ingredients and blend well.
3. Stir in whole wheat flour.
4. Shape into 1 inch balls and place on un-greased cookie sheet, 2 inches apart.
5. Flatten each cookie slightly with a fork.
6. Combine sugar and cinnamon and sprinkle over each cookie.
7. Decorate with M&M's or pecans. (optional)
8. Bake in pre-heated oven for 8 to 10 minutes or until light golden brown.

Makes a great gift!

**Note:** You can replace 1 C sugar, granulated with 1 C Vanilla Sugar; omit vanilla.

www.ingramcontent.com/pod-product-compliance
Lightning Source LLC
Chambersburg PA
CBHW050457290526
45786CB00006B/2337